EASY SOUS VIDE RECIPES

2021

FLAVORFUL RECIPES FOR ABSOLUTE BEGINNERS

ERIC FISHER

Table of Contents

Mustard & Honey Marinated Rack of Lamb

Prep + Cook Time: 1 hour 10 minutes | Servings: 4

Ingredients

1 rack of lamb, trimmed

3 tbsp honey

2 tbsp Dijon mustard

1 tsp sherry vinegar

Salt to taste

2 tbsp avocado oil

Chopped red onion

Directions

Prepare a water bath and place the Sous Vide in it. Set to 135 F. Combine well all the ingredients, except the lamb. Glaze the lamb with the mixture and place in a vacuum-sealable bag. Release air by the water displacement method, seal and submerge the bag in the water bath. Cook for 1 hour.

Once the timer has stopped, remove the lamb and transfer to a plate. Reserve the cooking juices. Heat the oil in a skillet over medium heat and sear the lamb for 2 minutes per side. Chop it and sprinkle with the cooking juices. Garnish with red onion.

Lamb Meatballs with a Yogurt Sauce

Prep + Cook Time: 2 hours 15 minutes | Servings: 2

Ingredients

½ pound ground lamb meat

¼ cup fresh parsley, chopped

¼ cup onion, minced

¼ cup toasted almond nuts, finely chopped

2 garlic cloves, minced

Salt to taste

2 tsp ground coriander

¼ tsp ground cinnamon

1 cup yogurt

½ cup diced cucumber

3 tbsp fresh mint, chopped

1 tsp lemon juice

¼ tsp cayenne pepper

Pitta bread

Directions

Prepare a water bath and place Sous Vide in it. Set to 134 F. Combine lamb, onion, almond, salt, garlic, cinnamon, and coriander. Make 20 balls and arrange them in a vacuum-sealable bag. Release air by the water displacement method, seal and submerge the bag in water bath. Cook for 120 minutes.

Meanwhile, prepare the sauce by mixing yogurt, mint, cucumber, cayenne, lemon juice, and 1 tbsp of salt. Once the timer has stopped, remove the balls and bake for 3-5 minutes. Top with the sauce and serve with pita bread.

Spicy Shoulder Lamb Rice

Prep + Cook Time: 24 hours 10 minutes | Servings: 2

Ingredients

1 lamb shoulder roast, boneless

1 tbsp olive oil

1 tbsp curry powder

2 tsp garlic salt

1 tsp coriander

1 tsp ground cumin

1 tsp dried red chili flakes

1 cup brown rice, cooked

Directions

Prepare a water bath and place the Sous Vide in it. Set to 158 F.

Combine the olive oil, garlic, salt, cumin, coriander, and chili flakes. Marinate the lamb. Place in a vacuum-sealable bag. Release air by the water displacement method, seal and submerge the bag in water bath. Cook for 24 hours.

Once done, remove the lamb and chop into slices. Serve with cooking juices over the rice.

Chili Lamb Steaks with Sesame Seed Topping

Prep + Cook Time: 3 hours 10 minutes | Servings: 2

Ingredients

2 lamb steaks

2 tbsp olive oil

Salt and black pepper to taste

2 tbsp avocado oil

1 tsp sesame seeds

Pinch of red pepper flakes

Directions

Prepare a water bath and place the Sous Vide in it. Set to 138 F. Place the lamb with olive oil in a vacuum-sealable bag. Release air by the water displacement method, seal and submerge the bag in water bath. Cook for 3 hours.

Once done, pat the lamb dry. Season with salt and pepper. Heat avocado oil in a skillet over high heat and sear the lamb. Chop into bites. Garnish with sesame seeds and pepper flakes.

Sweet Lamb with Mustard Sauce

Prep + Cook Time: 1 hour 10 minutes | Servings: 4

Ingredients

1 lamb of rack, trimmed

3 tbsp runny honey

2 tbsp Dijon mustard

1 tsp sherry wine vinegar

Salt to taste

2 tbsp avocado oil

1 tbsp thyme

Toasted mustard seeds for garnish

Chopped green onion

Directions

Prepare a water bath and place the Sous Vide in it. Set to 135 F. Combine all the ingredients, except the lamb. Place the lamb in a vacuum-sealable bag. Release air by the water displacement method, seal and submerge the bag in the water bath. Cook for 1 hour. Once the timer has stopped, remove the lamb and transfer to a plate.

Heat the oil in a frying pan over high heat and sear the lamb for 2 minutes each side. Chop and top with cooking juices. Garnish with green onion and toasted mustard seeds.

Lemon Mint Lamb

Prep + Cook Time: 2 hours 15 minutes | Servings: 2

Ingredients

1 rack of lamb

Salt and black pepper to taste

2 sprigs fresh rosemary

¼ cup olive oil

2 cups fresh lima beans, shelled, blanched and peeled

1 tbsp lemon juice

1 tbsp fresh chives, minced

1 tbsp fresh parsley, minced

1 tbsp fresh mint

1 garlic clove, minced

Directions

Prepare a water bath and place the Sous Vide in it. Set to 125 F. Season the lamb with salt and pepper and place in a vacuum-sealable bag. Release air by the water displacement method, seal and submerge the bag in water bath. Cook for 2 hours.

Once the timer has stopped, remove the lamb and pat dry. Heat 1 tbsp of olive oil in a grill over high heat and sear the seasoned lamb for 3 minutes. Set aside and allow chilling.

For the salad, combine the lima beans, lemon juice, parsley, chives, mint, garlic, and 3 tbsp of olive oil. Season with salt and pepper. Cut the lamb into chops and serve with lima beans salad.

Lemon Lamb Chops with Chimichurri Sauce

Prep + Cook Time: 2 hours 15 minutes | Servings: 4

Ingredients

4 lamb shoulder chops

2 tbsp avocado oil

Salt and black pepper to taste

1 cup firmly packed fresh parsley, chopped

2 tbsp fresh oregano

1 clove garlic, finely minced

1 tbsp champagne vinegar

1 tbsp lemon juice

1 tbsp smoked paprika

¼ tsp crushed red pepper flakes

1/3 cup salted butter, soft

Directions

Prepare a water bath and place Sous Vide in it. Set to 132 F. Season the lamb with salt and pepper and place in a vacuum-sealable bag. Release air by the water displacement method, seal and submerge the bag in the water bath. Cook for 2 hours.

Combine well in a bowl, the parsley, garlic, oregano, champagne vinegar, paprika, lemon juice, red pepper flakes, black pepper, salt, and soft butter. Allow chilling in the fridge.

Once the timer has stopped, remove the lamb and pat dry. Season with salt and pepper. Heat avocado oil in a skillet over high heat and sear the lamb for a few minutes on all sides. Top with butter dressing, and serve.

Lamb Shank with Veggies & Sweet Sauce

Prep + Cook Time: 48 hours 45 minutes | Servings: 4

Ingredients

4 lamb shanks

2 tbsp oil

2 cups all-purpose flour

1 red onion, sliced

4 garlic cloves, smashed and peeled

4 carrots, medium diced

4 stalks celery, medium diced

3 tbsp tomato paste

½ cup sherry wine vinegar

1 cup red wine

¾ cup honey

1 cup beef stock

4 sprigs fresh rosemary

2 bay leaves

Salt and black pepper to taste

Directions

Prepare a water bath and place the Sous Vide in it. Set to 155 F.

Heat oil in a skillet over high heat. Season the shanks with salt, pepper and flour. Sear until golden brown. Set aside. Reduce the heat and cook the onion, carrots, garlic, and celery for 10 minutes. Season with salt and pepper. Stir in tomato paste and cook for 1 more minute. Add in vinegar, stock, wine, honey, bay leaves. Cook for 2 minutes.

Place the veggies, sauce and lambs in a vacuum-sealable bag. Release air by the water displacement method, seal and submerge the bag in the water bath. Cook for 48 hours.

Once the timer has stopped, remove the shanks and dry it. Reserve the cooking juices. Sear the shanks for 5 minutes until golden. Heat a saucepan over high and pour in cooking juices. Cook until reduced, for10 minutes. Transfer the shanks to a plate and drizzle with the sauce to serve.

Pancetta & Lamb Stew

Prep + Cook Time: 24 hours 25 minutes | Servings: 6

Ingredients

2 pounds boneless lamb shoulder, cubed

4 oz pancetta, cut into strips

1 cup red wine

2 tbsp tomato paste

1 cup beef stock

4 large shallots, quartered

4 baby carrots, chopped

4 stalks celery, chopped

3 cloves garlic, smashed

1 pound fingerling potatoes, cut lengthwise

4 oz dried Portobello mushrooms

3 sprigs fresh rosemary

3 sprigs fresh thyme

Salt and black pepper to taste

Directions

Prepare a water bath and place the Sous Vide in it. Set to 146 F.

Heat a skillet over high heat and cook the pancetta until browned. Set aside. Season the lamb with salt and pepper and sear in the same skillet; set aside. Pour in wine and stock, and cook for 5 minutes.

Place wine mix, lamb, pancetta, searing juices, veggies and herbs in a vacuum-sealable bag. Release air by the water displacement method, seal and submerge the bag in the water bath. Cook for 24 hours.

Once the timer has stopped, remove the bag and transfer cooking juices to a hot saucepan over medium heat and cook for 15 minutes Stir in the lamb to sear for a few minutes and serve.

Peppery Lemon Lamb Chops with Papaya Chutney

Prep + Cook Time: 1 hour 15 minutes | Servings: 4

Ingredients

8 lamb chops

2 tbsp olive oil

½ tsp Garam Masala

¼ tsp lemon pepper

Dash of garlic pepper

Salt and black pepper to taste

½ cup yogurt

¼ cup fresh cilantro, chopped

2 tbsp papaya chutney

1 tbsp curry powder

1 tbsp onion, finely chopped

Chopped cilantro for garnish

Directions

Prepare a water bath and place the Sous Vide in it. Set to 138 F. Brush the chops with olive oil and top with Garam Masala, lemon pepper, garlic powder, salt, and pepper. Place in a vacuum-sealable bag. Release air by the water displacement method, seal and submerge the bag in the water bath. Cook for 1 hour.

Meanwhile, prepare the sauce by mixing yogurt, papaya chutney, cilantro, curry powder, and onion. Transfer to a plate. Once the timer has stopped, remove the lamb and dry. Heat the remaining oil in a skillet over medium heat and sear the lamb for 30 seconds per side. Strain with a baking sheet. Serve the chops with the yogurt sauce. Garnish with cilantro.

Spicy Lamb Kebabs

Prep + Cook Time: 2 hours 20 minutes | Servings: 4

Ingredients

1 pound leg lamb, boneless, cubed

2 tbsp chili paste

1 tbsp olive oil

Salt to taste

1 tsp cumin

1 tsp coriander

½ tsp black pepper

Greek yogurt

Fresh mint leaves for serving

Directions

Prepare a water bath and place the Sous Vide in it. Set to 134 F. Combine all the ingredients and place in a vacuum-sealable bag. Release air by the water displacement method, seal and submerge the bag in the water bath. Cook for 2 hours.

Once the timer has stopped, remove the lamb and dry it. Transfer the lamb to a grill and cook for 5 minutes. Set aside and allow resting for 5 minutes. Serve with Greek yogurt and mint.

Herby Lamb with Veggies

Prep + Cook Time: 48 hours 30 minutes | Servings: 8)

Ingredients

2 lamb shanks, bone-in

1 can diced tomatoes with juice

1 cup veal stock

1 cup onion, finely diced

½ cup celery, finely diced

½ cup carrot, finely diced

½ cup red wine

2 sprigs fresh rosemary

Salt and black pepper to taste

1 tsp ground coria

1 tsp ground cumin

1 teaspoon thyme

Directions

Prepare a water bath and place the Sous Vide in it. Set to 149 F.

Combine all the ingredients and place in a vacuum-sealable bag. Release air by the water displacement method, seal and submerge the bag in the water bath. Cook for 48 hours.

Once the timer has stopped, remove the shanks and transfer to a plate and allow cooling for 48 hours. Clean the lamb removing the bones and the fat then chop into bites. Transfer the no-fat cooking juices and bites lambs to a saucepan. Cook for 10 minutes over high heat until the sauce thickens. Serve.

Garlic Rack of Lamb

Prep + Cook Time: 1 hour 30 minutes | Servings: 4

Ingredients

2 tbsp butter

2 racks of lamb, frenched

1 tbsp olive oil

1 tbsp sesame oil

4 garlic cloves, minced

4 fresh basil sprigs, halved

Salt and black pepper to taste

Directions

Prepare a water bath and place the Sous Vide in it. Set to 130 F. Season the rack lamb with salt and pepper. Place in a large vacuum-sealable bag. Release air by the water displacement method, seal and submerge the bag in the water bath. Cook for 1 hour and 15 minutes.

Once the timer has stopped, remove the rack and pat dry with kitchen towel. Heat sesame oil in a skillet over high heat and sear the rack for 1 minute per side. Set aside.

Put 1 tbsp of butter in the skillet and add in half of garlic and half of basil. Top over the rack. Sear the rack for 1 minute. Turn around and pour in more butter. Repeat the process for all racks. Cut into pieces and serve 4 pieces in each plate.

Herb Crusted Lamb Rack

Prep + Cook Time: 3 hours 30 minutes | Servings: 6

Ingredients:

<u>Lamb Rack:</u>

3 large racks of lamb

Salt and black pepper to taste

1 sprig rosemary

2 tbsp olive oil

<u>Herb Crust:</u>

2 tbsp fresh rosemary leaves

½ cup macadamia nuts

2 tbsp Dijon mustard

½ cup fresh parsley

2 tbsp fresh thyme leaves

2 tbsp lemon zest

2 cloves garlic

2 Egg whites

Directions:

Make a water bath, place the Sous Vide in it, and set to 140 F.

Pat dry the lamb using a paper towel and rub the meat with salt and black pepper. Place a pan over medium heat and add in olive oil. Once heated, sear the lamb on both sides for 2 minutes; set aside.

Place in garlic and rosemary, toast for 2 minutes and place the lamb over. Let lamb absorb the flavors for 5 minutes.

Place lamb, garlic, and rosemary in a vacuum-sealable bag, release air by the water displacement method and seal the bag. Submerge the bag in the water bath.

Set the timer to cook for 3 hours. Once the timer has stopped, remove the bag, unseal it and take out the lamb. Whisk the egg whites and set aside.

Blend the remaining listed herb crust ingredients using a blender and set aside. Pat dry the lamb using a paper towel and brush with the egg whites. Dip into the herb mixture and coat graciously.

Place the lamb racks with crust side up on a baking sheet. Bake in an oven for 15 minutes. Gently slice each cutlet using a sharp knife. Serve with a side of pureed vegetables.

Popular South African Lamb & Cherry Kebabs

Prep + Cook Time: 8 hours 40 minutes | Servings: 6

Ingredients

¾ cup white wine vinegar

½ cup dry red wine

2 onions, chopped

4 garlic cloves, minced

Zest of 2 lemons

6 tbsp brown sugar

2 tbsp caraway seeds, crushed

1 tbsp cherry jam

1 tbsp cornflour

1 tbsp curry powder

1 tbsp grated ginger

2 tsp salt

1 tsp allspice

1 tsp ground cinnamon

4½ pounds lamb shoulder, cubed

1 tbsp butter

6 pearl onions, peeled and halved

12 dried cherries, halved

2 tbsp olive oi

Directions

Prepare a water bath and place the Sous Vide in it. Set to 141 F.

Combine well the vinegar, red wine, onions, garlic, lemon zest, brown sugar, caraway seeds, cherry jam, corn flour, curry powder, ginger, salt, allspice, and cinnamon.

Place the lamb in a large vacuum-sealable bag. Release air by the water displacement method, seal and submerge the bag in the water bath. Cook for 8 hours. Before 20 minutes to the end, heat the butter in a saucepan and sauté the pearl onions for 8 minutes until softened. Set aside and allow to cool.

Once the timer has stopped, remove the lamb and pat dry with kitchen towel. Reserve the cooking juices and transfer into a saucepan over medium heat and cook for 10 minutes until reduced by half. Fill the skewer with all kebab ingredients and roll them. Heat olive oil in a grill over high heat and cook the kebabs for 45 seconds per side.

Bell Pepper & Lamb Curry

Prep + Cook Time: 30 hours 30 minutes | Servings: 4

Ingredients

2 tbsp butter

2 bell peppers, chopped

3 garlic cloves, minced

1 tsp turmeric

1 tsp ground cumin

1 tsp paprika

1 tsp grated fresh ginger

½ tsp salt

2 cardamom pods

2 fresh thyme sprigs

2¼ pounds boneless lamb meat, cubed

1 large onion, chopped

3 tomatoes, chopped

1 tsp allspice

2 tbsp Greek yogurt

1 tbsp chopped fresh cilantro

Directions

Prepare a water bath and place the Sous Vide in it. Set to 179 F. Combine 1 tbsp of butter, bell peppers, 2 garlic cloves, turmeric, cumin, paprika, ginger, salt, cardamom, and thyme. Place the lamb in a vacuum-sealable bag with the butter mixture. Release air by the water displacement method, seal and submerge the bag in the water bath. Cook for 30 hours.

Once the timer has stopped, remove the bag and set aside. Heat the butter in a saucepan over high heat. Add in onion and cook for 4 minutes. Add the remaining garlic and cook for 1 minute more. Reduce the heat and place in tomatoes and allspice. Cook for 2 minutes. Pour in yogurt, lamb and the cooking juices. Cook for 10-15 minutes. Garnish with cilantro.

Goat Cheese Lamb Ribs

Prep + Cook Time: 4 hours 10 minutes | Servings: 2

Ingredients:

Ribs:

2 half racks lamb ribs

2 tbsp vegetable oil

1 clove garlic, minced

2 tbsp rosemary leaves, chopped

1 tbsp fennel pollen

Salt and black pepper to taste

½ tsp cayenne pepper

To Garnish:

8 oz goat cheese, crumbled

2 oz roasted walnuts, chopped

3 tbsp parsley, chopped

Directions:

Make a water bath, place the Sous Vide in it, and set to 134 F. Mix the listed lamb ingredients except for the lamb. Pat dry the lamb using a kitchen towel and rub with the spice mixture. Place the meat in a vacuum-sealable bag, release air by the water displacement method, seal and submerge the bag in the water bath. Set the timer for 4 hours.

Once the timer has stopped, remove the lamb. Preheat a grill over high heat and add in oil. Sear the lamb until golden brown. Cut the ribs between the bones. Garnish with goat cheese, walnuts and parsley. Serve with a hot sauce dip.

Lamb Shoulder

Prep + Cook Time: 4 hours 10 minutes | Servings: 3

Ingredients:

1 pound lamb shoulder, deboned

Salt and black pepper to taste

2 tbsp olive oil

1 garlic clove, crushed

1 sprig thyme

1 sprig sosemary

Directions:

Prepare a water bath and place the Sous Vide in it. Set to 145 F. Pat dry the lamb shoulders using a paper towel and rub with pepper and salt.

Place the lamb and the remaining listed ingredients in a vacuum-sealable bag. Release air by the water displacement method, seal and submerge the bag in the water bath. Set the timer for 4 hours.

Once done, remove the bag and transfer the lamb shoulders to baking dish. Strain the juices into a saucepan and cook over medium heat for 2 minutes. Preheat a grill for 10 minutes and grill the shoulder until golden brown and crispy. Serve the lamb shoulder and sauce with a side of buttered greens.

Jalapeño Lamb Roast

Prep + Cook Time: 3 hours | Servings: 6

Ingredients:

1 ½ tbsp canola oil

1 tbsp black mustard seeds

1 tsp cumin seeds

Salt and black pepper to taste

4 lb butterflied lamb leg

½ cup mint leaves, chopped

½ cup cilantro leaves, chopped

1 shallot, minced

1 clove garlic, minced

2 red jalapenos, minced

1 tbsp red wine vinegar

1 ½ tbsp olive oil

Directions:

Place a skillet over low heat on a stove top. Add ½ tablespoon of olive oil; once it has heated, add in cumin and mustard seeds and cook for 1 minute. Turn off heat and transfer seeds to a bowl. Sprinkle with salt and black pepper. Mix. Spread half of the spice mixture inside the lamb leg and roll it. Secure with a butcher's twine at 1- inch intervals.

Season with salt and pepper and massage. Spread half of the spice mixture evenly over of lamb leg, then carefully roll it back up. Make a water bath and place Sous Vide in it. Set to 145 F. Place the lamb leg in vacuum-sealable bag, release air by the water displacement method, seal and submerge it in the water bath. Set the timer for 2 hours 45 minutes and cook.

Make the sauce; add to the cumin mustard mixture shallot, cilantro, garlic, red wine vinegar, mint, and red chili. Mix and season with salt and pepper. Set aside. Once the timer has stopped, remove and unseal the bag. Remove the lamb and pat dry using a paper towel.

Add canola oil to a cast iron, preheat over high heat for 10 minutes. Place in lamb and sear to brown on both sides. Remove twine and slice lamb. Serve with sauce.

Thyme & Sage Grilled Lamb Chops

Prep + Cook Time: 3 hours 20 minutes | Servings: 6

Ingredients

6 tbsp butter

4 tbsp dry white wine

4 tbsp chicken broth

4 fresh thyme sprigs

2 garlic cloves, minced

1½ tsp chopped fresh sage

1½ tsp cumin

6 lamb chops

Salt and black pepper to taste

2 tbsp olive oil

Directions

Prepare a water bath and place the Sous Vide in it. Set to 134 F.

Heat a pot over medium heat and combine butter, white wine, broth, thyme, garlic, cumin, and sage. Cook for 5 minutes. Allow to cool. Season the lamb with salt and pepper. Place in three vacuum-sealable bags with the butter mixture. Release air by the water displacement method, seal and submerge the bags in the water bath. Cook for 3 hours.

Once done, remove the lamb and pat dry with kitchen towel. Brush the chops with olive oil. Heat a skillet over high heat and sear the lamb for 45 seconds per side. Allow to rest for 5 minutes.

Lamb Chops with Basil Chimichurri

Prep + Cook Time: 3 hours 40 minutes | Servings: 4

Ingredients:

Lamb Chops:

3 lamb racks, frenched

3 cloves garlic, crushed

Salt and black pepper to taste

Basil Chimichurri:

1 ½ cups fresh basil, finely chopped

2 banana shallots, diced

3 cloves garlic, minced

1 tsp red pepper flakes

½ cup olive oil

3 tbsp red wine vinegar

Salt and black pepper to taste

Directions:

Prepare a water bath and place the Sous Vide in it. Set to 140 F. Pat dry the racks with a kitchen towel and rub with pepper and salt. Place meat and garlic in a vacuum-sealable bag, release air by water displacement method and seal the bag. Submerge the bag in the water bath. Set the timer for 2 hours and cook.

Make the basil chimichurri: mix all the listed ingredients in a bowl. Cover with cling film and refrigerate for 1 hour 30 minutes. Once the timer has stopped, remove the bag and open it. Remove the lamb and pat dry using a paper towel. Sear with a torch to golden brown. Pour the basil chimichurri on the lamb. Serve with a side of steamed greens.

Savory Harissa Lamb Kabobs

Prep + Cook Time: 2 hours 30 minutes | Servings: 10

Ingredients

3 tbsp olive oil

4 tsp red wine vinegar

2 tbsp chili paste

2 garlic cloves, minced

1½ tsp ground cumin

1½ tsp ground coriander

1 tsp hot paprika

Salt to taste

1½ pounds boneless lamb shoulder, cubed

1 cucumber, peeled and chopped

Zest and juice of ½ lemon

1 cup Greek-style yogurt

Directions

Prepare a water bath and place the Sous Vide in it. Set to 134 F. Combine 2 tbsp of olive oil, vinegar, chili, garlic, cumin, coriander, paprika, and salt. Place the lamb and sauce in a vacuum-sealable bag. Release air by water displacement method, seal and submerge the bag in the bath. Cook for 2 hours.

Once the timer has stopped, remove the lamb and pat dry with kitchen towel. Discard cooking juices. Mix the cucumber, lemon zest and juice, yogurt, and pressed garlic in a small bowl. Set aside. Fill the skewer with the lamb and roll it.

Heat the oil in a skillet over high heat and cook the skewer for 1-2 minutes per side. Top with the lemon-garlic sauce and serve.

Sweet Mustard Pork with Crispy Onions

Prep + Cook Time: 48 hours 40 minutes | Servings: 6

Ingredients

1 tbsp ketchup

4 tbsp honey mustard

2 tbsp soy sauce

2¼ pounds pork shoulder

1 large sweet onion, cut into thin rings

2 cups milk

1½ cups all-purpose flour

2 tsp granulated onion powder

1 tsp paprika

Salt and black pepper to taste

4 cups vegetable oil, for frying

Directions

Prepare a water bath and place the Sous Vide in it. Set to 159 F.

Combine well the mustard, soy sauce and ketchup to make a paste. Brush the pork with the sauce and place in a vacuum-sealable bag. Release air by the water displacement method, seal and submerge the bag in the water bath. Cook for 48 hours.

To make the onions: separate the onion rings in a bowl. Pour the milk over them and allow to chill for 1 hour. Combine the flour, onion powder paprika, and a pinch of salt and pepper.

Heat the oil in a skillet to 375 F. Drain the onions and deepen in the flour mix. Shake well and transfer into the skillet. Fry them for 2 minutes or until gets crispy. Transfer to a baking sheet and pat dry with kitchen towel. Repeat the process with the remaining onions.

Once the timer has stopped, remove the pork and transfer to a cutting board and pull the pork until it is shredded. Reserve cooking juices and transfer into a saucepan hot over medium heat and cook for 5 minutes until reduced. Top the pork with the sauce and garnish with the crispy onions to serve.

Delicious Basil & Lemon Pork Chops

Prep + Cook Time: 1 hour 15 minutes | Servings: 4

Ingredients

4 tbsp butter

4 boneless pork rib chops

Salt and black pepper to taste

Zest and juice of 1 lemon

2 garlic cloves, smashed

2 bay leaves

1 fresh basil sprig

Directions

Prepare a water bath and place the Sous Vide in it. Set to 141 F Season the chops with salt and pepper.

Place the chops with the lemon zest and juice, garlic, bay leaves, basil, and 2 tbsp of butter in a vacuum-sealable bag. Release air by the water displacement method, seal and submerge the bag in the water bath. Cook for 1 hour.

Once the timer has stopped, remove the chops and pat dry with kitchen towel. Reserve the herbs. Heat the remaining butter in a skillet over medium heat and sear for 1-2 minutes per side.

Baby Ribs with Chinese Sauce

Prep + Cook Time: 4 hours 25 minutes | Servings: 4

Ingredients

1/3 cup hoisin sauce

1/3 cup dark soy sauce

1/3 cup sugar

3 tbsp honey

3 tbsp white vinegar

1 tbsp fermented bean paste

2 tsp sesame oil

2 crushed garlic cloves

1-inch piece fresh grated ginger

1 ½ tsp five-spice powder

Salt to taste

½ tsp fresh ground black pepper

3 pounds baby back ribs

Cilantro leaves for serving

Directions

Prepare a water bath and place the Sous Vide in it. Set to 168 F.

Combine in a bowl hoisin sauce, dark soy sauce, sugar, white vinegar, honey, bean paste, sesame oil, five-spice powder, salt, ginger, white and black pepper. Reserve 1/3 of the mixture and allow chilling.

Brush the ribs with the mixture and share among 3 vacuum-sealable bag. Release air by the water displacement method, seal and submerge the bags in the water bath. Cook for 4 hours.

Preheat the oven to 400 F. Once the timer has stopped, remove the ribs and brush with the remaining mixture. Transfer to a baking tray and put in the oven. Bake for 3 minutes. Take out and allow resting for 5 minutes. Cut the rack and top with cilantro.

Pork & Bean Stew

Prep + Cook Time: 7 hours 20 minutes | Servings: 8)

Ingredients

2 tbsp vegetable oil

1 tbsp butter

1 trimmed pork loin, cubed

Salt and black pepper to taste

2 cups frozen pearl onions

2 large parsnips, chopped

2 minced cloves garlic

2 tbsp all-purpose flour

1 cup dry white wine

2 cups chicken stock

1 can white beans, drained and rinsed

4 fresh rosemary sprigs

2 bay leaves

Directions

Prepare a water bath and place the Sous Vide in it. Set to 138 F.

Heat a non-stick pan over high heat with butter and oil. Add the pork. Season with pepper and salt. Cook for 7 minutes. Put in onions and cook for 5 minutes. Mix the garlic and wine until bubble. Stir in beans, rosemary, stock, and bay leaves. Remove from the heat.

Place the pork in a vacuum-sealable bag. Release air by the water displacement method, seal and submerge the bag in the water bath. Cook for 7 hours. Once the timer has stopped, remove the bag and transfer into a bowl. Garnish with rosemary.

Jerk Pork Ribs

Prep + Cook Time: 20 hours 10 minutes | Servings: 6

Ingredients:

5 lb (2) baby back pork ribs, full racks

½ cup jerk seasoning mix

Directions:

Make a water bath, place Sous Vide in it, and set to 145 F. Cut the racks into halves and season them with half of jerk seasoning. Place the racks in separate vacuum-sealable racks. Release air by the water displacement method, seal and submerge the bags in the water bath. Set the timer to 20 hours.

Cover the water bath with a bag to reduce evaporation and add water every 3 hours to avoid the water drying out. Once the timer has stopped, remove and unseal the bag. Transfer the ribs to a foiled baking sheet and preheat a broiler to high. Rub the ribs with the remaining jerk seasoning and place them in the broiler. Broil for 5 minutes. Slice into single ribs.

Balsamic Pork Chops

Prep + Cook Time: 1 hour 15 minutes | Servings: 5

Ingredients:

2 pounds pork chops

3 garlic cloves, crushed

½ tsp dried basil

½ tsp dried thyme

¼ cup balsamic vinegar

Salt and black pepper to taste

3 tbsp extra virgin olive oil

Directions:

Prepare a water bath, place Sous Vide in it, and set to 158 F. Season the pork chops generously with salt and pepper; set aside.

In a small bowl, combine vinegar with 1 tbsp of olive oil, thyme, basil, and garlic. Stir well and spread the mixture evenly over meat. Place in a large vacuum-sealable bag and seal it. Submerge the sealed bag in the water bath and cook for for 1 hour.

Once the timer has stopped, take the pork chops out of the bag, and pat them dry. Heat the remaining olive oil in a medium size pan over high heat. Sear the chops for one minute per side, or until golden brown. Add in cooking juices and simmer for 3-4 minutes or until thickened.

Boneless Pork Ribs with Coconut-Peanut Sauce

Prep + Cook Time: 8 hours 30 minutes | Servings: 3

Ingredients:

½ cup coconut milk

2 ½ tbsp peanut butter

2 tbsp soy sauce

1 tbsp sugar

3 inches fresh lemongrass

1 ½ tbsp pepper sauce

1 ½ inch ginger, peeled

3 cloves garlic

2 ½ tsp sesame oil

13 oz boneless pork ribs

Directions:

Prepare a water bath and place Sous Vide in it. Set to 135 F. Blend all listed ingredients in a blender, except for the pork ribs and cilantro, until a smooth paste is obtained.

Place the ribs in a vacuum-sealable bag and add in sauce. Release air by the water displacement method and seal the bag. Place in the water bath and set the timer for 8 hours.

Once the timer has stopped, take the bag out, unseal it and remove the ribs. Transfer to a plate and keep it warm. Put a skillet over medium heat and pour in the sauce of the bag. Bring to boil for 5 minutes, reduce the heat, and simmer for 12 minutes.

Add the ribs and coat with the sauce. Simmer for 6 minutes. Serve with a side of steamed greens.

Lime and Garlic Pork Tenderloin

Prep + Cook Time: 2 hours 15 minutes | Servings: 2

Ingredients:

2 tbsp garlic powder

2 tbsp ground cumin

2 tbsp dried thyme

2 tbsp dried rosemary

1 pinch lime sea salt

2 (3-lb) pork tenderloin, silver skin removed

2 tbsp olive oil

3 tbsp unsalted butter

Directions:

Make a water bath, place Sous Vide in it, and set to 140 F. Add the cumin, garlic powder, thyme, lime salt, rosemary, and lime salt to a bowl and mix evenly. Brush the pork with olive oil and rub with salt and cumin herb mixture.

Put the pork into two separate vacuum-sealable bags. Release air by the water displacement method and seal the bags. Submerge in the water bath and set the timer for 2 hours.

Once the timer has stopped, remove and unseal the bag. Remove the pork and pat dry using a paper towel. Discard the juice in the bag. Preheat a cast iron pan over high heat and add in butter. Place in pork and sear to golden brown. Let the pork rest on a cutting board. Cut them into 2-inch medallions.

BBQ Pork Ribs

Prep + Cook Time: 1 hour 10 minutes | Servings: 4

Ingredients:

1 lb pork ribs

1 tsp garlic powder

Salt and black pepper to taste

1 cup BBQ sauce

Directions:

Make a water bath, place Sous Vide in it, and set to 140 F. Rub salt and pepper on the pork ribs, place in a vacuum-sealable bag, release air and seal it. Put in the water and set the timer to 1 hour.

Once the timer has stopped, remove and unseal the bag. Remove ribs and coat with BBQ sauce. Set aside. Preheat a grill. Once it is hot, sear the ribs all around for 5 minutes. Serve with a dip of choice.

Maple Tenderloin with Sautéed Apple

Prep + Cook Time: 2 hours 20 minutes | Servings: 4

Ingredients

1 pound pork tenderloin

1 tbsp fresh rosemary, chopped

1 tbsp maple syrup

1 tsp black pepper

Salt to taste

1 tbsp olive oil

1 apple, diced

1 thinly sliced small shallot

¼ cup vegetable broth

½ tsp apple cider

Directions

Prepare a water bath and place the Sous Vide in it. Set to 135 F. Remove the skin from the tenderloin and cut by the half. Combine the rosemary, maple syrup, ground pepper, and 1 tbsp of salt. Sprinkle over the tenderloin. Place in a vacuum-sealable bag. Release air by the water displacement method, seal and submerge the bag in the water bath. Cook for 2 hours.

Once the timer has stopped, remove the bag and dry it. Reserve the cooking juices. Heat olive oil in a skillet over medium heat and sear the tenderloin for 5 minutes. Set aside.

Low the heat and put in apple, rosemary springs, and shallot. Season with salt and sauté for 2-3 minutes until golden. Add in vinegar, broth, and cooking juices. Simmer for 3-5 minutes more. Cut the tenderloin into medallions and serve with the apple mix.

BBQ Beef Brisket

Prep + Cook Time: 48 hours 15 minutes | Servings: 8

Ingredients:

1 ½ pound beef brisket

Salt and black pepper to taste

1 tbsp olive oil

1 tbsp garlic powder

Directions:

Prepare a water bath and place the Sous Vide in it. Set to 150 F. Rub the salt, pepper and garlic powder over the meat and place it in a vacuum-sealable bag. Release air by the water displacement method, seal and submerge in the water bath. Set the timer for 48 hours. After 2 days, heat the olive oil in a pan over medium heat. Remove the beef from the bag and sear all sides.

Sirloin Steaks with Mushroom Cream Sauce

Prep + Cook Time: 1 hour 20 minutes | Servings: 3

Ingredients:

3 (6-oz) boneless sirloin steaks

Salt and black pepper to taste

4 tsp unsalted butter

1 tbsp olive oil

6 oz white mushrooms, quartered

2 large shallots, minced

2 cloves garlic, minced

½ cup beef stock

½ cup heavy cream

2 tsp mustard sauce

Thinly sliced scallions for garnishing

Directions:

Prepare a water bath, place Sous Vide in it, and set to 135 ºF. Season the beef with pepper and salt and place them in a 3 separate vacuum-sealable bag. Add 1 teaspoon of butter to each bag. Release air by the water displacement method, seal and submerge the bag in the water bath. Set to 45 minutes.

Ten minutes before the timer stops, heat oil and the remaining butter in a skillet over medium heat. Once the timer has stopped, remove and unseal the bag. Remove the beef, pat dry, and place in the skillet. Reserve the juices in the bags. Sear on each side for 1 minute and transfer to cutting board. Slice and set aside.

In the same skillet, add the shallots and mushrooms. Cook for 10 minutes and add the garlic. Cook for 1 minute. Add the stock and reserved juices. Simmer for 3 minutes. Add in heavy cream, bring to a boil on high heat and reduce to lower heat after 5 minutes. Turn the heat off and stir in the mustard sauce. Place the steak on a plate, top with mushroom sauce and garnish with scallions.

Prime Rib with Celery Herb Crust

Prep + Cook Time: 5 hours 15 minutes | Servings: 3

Ingredients:

1 ½ lb rib eye steak, bone in

Salt and black pepper to taste

½ tsp pink pepper

½ tbsp celery seeds, dried

1 tbsp garlic powder

2 sprigs rosemary, minced

2 cups beef stock

1 egg white

Directions:

Rub salt on the meat and marinate for 1 hour. Make a water bath, place Sous Vide in it, and set to 130 F. Place beef in a vacuum-sealable bag, release air by the water displacement method and seal the bag. Submerge the bag in the water bath. Set the timer for 4 hours and cook. Once ready, remove the beef and pat dry; set aside.

Mix the black pepper powder, pink pepper powder, celery seeds, garlic powder, and rosemary. Brush the beef with the egg white. Dip the beef in the celery seed mixture to coat graciously. Place in a baking sheet and bake in an oven for 15 minutes. Remove and allow to cool on a cutting board.

Gently slice the beef, cutting against the bone. Pour liquid in a vacuum bag and beef broth in a pan and bring to boil over medium heat. Discard floating fat or solids. Place beef slices on a plate and drizzle sauce over it. Serve with a side of steamed green vegetables.

Beef Steak with Shallots and Parsley

Prep + Cook Time: 1 hour 15 minutes | Servings: 4

Ingredients:

2 pounds beef steak, sliced

2 tbsp Dijon mustard

3 tbsp olive oil

1 tbsp fresh parsley leaves, finely chopped

1 tsp fresh rosemary, finely chopped

1 tbsp shallot, finely chopped

½ tsp dried thyme

1 garlic clove, crushed

Directions:

Prepare a water bath and place Sous Vide in it. Set to 136 F.

In a small bowl, combine Dijon mustard, olive oil, parsley, rosemary, shallot, thyme, and garlic. Rub the meat with this mixture and place in a vacuum-sealable bag. Release air by the water displacement method, seal and submerge the bag in the water bath. Set the timer for 1 hour. Serve with salad.

Shredded BBQ Roast

Prep + Cook Time: 14 hours 20 minutes | Servings: 3

Ingredients:

1 pound beef chuck roast

2 tbsp BBQ seasoning

Directions:

Make a water bath, place the Sous Vide in it, and set to 165 F.

Preheat a grill. Pat dry the meat using a paper towel and rub with BBQ seasoning. Set aside for 15 minutes. Place meat in vacuum-sealable bag, release air by water displacement method and seal bag.

Submerge in the water bath. Set the timer for 14 hours and cook. Once the timer has stopped, remove the bag and unseal it. Remove the meat and shred it. Serve.

Simple Corned Beef

Prep + Cook Time: 5 hours 10 minutes | Servings: 4

Ingredients:

15 ounces beef brisket

1 tbsp salt

¼ cup beef stock

1 tsp paprika

1 cup beer

2 onions, sliced

½ tsp oregano

1 tsp cayenne pepper

Directions:

Prepare a water bath and place Sous Vide in it. Set to 138 F. Cut the beef into 4 pieces. Place in separate vacuum-sealable bags. Whisk beer, stock and spices in a bowl. Stir in the onions. Divide the mixture between the bags.

Release air by the water displacement method, seal and submerge the bag in water bath. Set the timer for 5 hours. Once the timer has stopped, remove the bag and tranfer to a plate.

Fire-Roasted Tomato Tenderloin

Prep + Cook Time: 2 hours 8 minutes | Servings: 4

Ingredients:

2 pounds center-cut beef tenderloin, 1-inch thick

1 cup fire-roasted tomatoes, chopped

Salt and black pepper to taste

3 tbsp of extra virgin olive oil

2 bay leaves, whole

3 tbsp of butter, unsalted

Directions:

Prepare a water bath, place Sous Vide in it, and set to 136 F. Thoroughly rinse the meat under the running water and pat dry with paper towels. Rub well with the olive oil and generously season with salt and pepper. Place in a large vacuum-sealable bag along with fire-roasted tomatoes and two bay leaves. Seal the bag, submerge in the water bath and cook for 2 hours.

Once done, remove the bags, place the meat on a baking sheet. Discard the cooking liquid. In a large skillet, melt the butter over medium heat. Add the tenderloin and sear for 2 minutes on each side. Serve with your favorite sauce and vegetables.

Sirloin Steak with Mashed Turnips

Prep + Cook Time: 1 hour 20 minutes | Servings: 4

Ingredients:

4 sirloin steaks

2 lbs of turnips, diced

Salt and black pepper to taste

4 tbsp butter

Olive oil for searing

Directions:

Make a water bath, place Sous Vide in it, and set it to 128 F. Season steaks with pepper and salt and place in a vacuum-sealable bag. Release air by the water displacement method, seal and submerge the bag in the water bath. Set the timer for 1 hour.

Place turnips in boiling water and cook until tender for about 10 minutes. Strain turnips and place in a mixing bowl. Add in butter and mash them. Season with pepper and salt.

Once the timer has stopped, remove and unseal the bags. Remove the steaks from the bag and pat dry. Season to taste. Sear the steaks in a pan with oil over medium heat for about 2 minutes on each side. Serve steaks with mashed turnips.

Flank Steak with Tomato Roast

Prep + Cook Time: 3 hours 30 minutes | Servings: 3

Ingredients:

1 lb flank steak

4 tbsp olive oil, divided into two

1 tbsp + 1 tsp italian seasoning

Salt and black pepper to taste

4 cloves garlic, 2 cloves crushed + 2 cloves whole

1 cup cherry tomatoes

1 tbsp balsamic vinegar

3 tbsp Parmesan cheese, grated

Directions:

Prepare a water bath, place Sous Vide in it, and set to 129 F. Place the steak in a vacuum-sealable bag. Add half of olive oil, Italian seasoning, black pepper, salt, and crushed garlic and rub gently.

Release air by the water displacement method and seal the bag. Submerge in the water bath. Set the timer for 3 hours and cook 10 minutes. Before the timer has stopped, preheat an oven to 400 F.

In a bowl, toss tomatoes with the remaining ingredients, except for the Parmesan cheese. Pour into a baking dish and place in the oven on the farthest rack from the fire. Bake for 15 minutes.

Once the timer has stopped, remove the bag, unseal and remove the steak. Transfer to a flat surface and sear both sides with a torch until golden brown. Let cool and slice thinly. Serve steak with tomato roast. Garnish with Parmesan cheese.

Beef Pear Steak

Prep + Cook Time: 3 hours 10 minutes | Servings: 3

Ingredients:

3 (6 oz) beef pear steaks

2 tbsp olive oil

4 tbsp unsalted butter

4 cloves garlic, crushed

4 sprigs fresh thyme

Directions:

Make a water bath, place the Sous Vide in it, and set to 135F. Season the beef with salt and place in 3 vacuum-sealable bags. Release air by the water displacement method and seal bags. Submerge in the water bath. Set the timer for 3 hours and cook.

Once the timer has stopped, remove the beef, pat dry, and season with pepper and salt. Warm oil in a skillet over medium heat until it starts to smoke. Add the steaks, butter, garlic, and thyme. Sear for 3 minutes on both sides. Baste with some more butter as you cook. Slice steaks into desired slices.

Beef Chuck Shoulder with Mushrooms

Prep + Cook Time: 6 hours 15 minutes | Servings: 3

Ingredients:

1 pound beef chuck shoulder

1 medium-sized carrot, sliced

1 large onion, chopped

¾ cup button mushrooms, sliced

1 cup beef stock

2 tbsp olive oil

4 garlic cloves, finely chopped

Salt and black pepper to taste

Directions:

Prepare a water bath and place the Sous Vide in it. Set to 136 F. Place beef chuck shoulder in a large vacuum-sealable bag along with sliced carrot, and half of the broth. Submerge the sealed bag in the water bath and cook for 6 hours. Once the timer has stopped, remove the meat from bag and pat dry.

In a pot, heat up the olive oil and put in onion and garlic. Stir-fry until translucent, for 3-4 minutes. Add beef shoulder, the remaining broth, 2 cups of water, mushrooms, salt, and pepper. Bring it to a boil and reduce the heat to minimum. Cook for an additional 5 minutes, stirring constantly.

Tomato Stuffed Mushrooms

Prep + Cook Time: 60 minutes | Servings: 4

Ingredients:

2 pounds Cremini mushrooms

1 yellow bell pepper, finely chopped

2 medium-sized tomatoes, peeled and finely chopped

2 spring onions, finely chopped

1 ¾ cup lean ground beef

3 tbsp olive oil

Salt and black pepper to taste

Directions:

Prepare a water bath and place the Sous Vide in it. Set to 131 F. Steam the mushrooms and set caps aside. Chop up the mushroom stems. Heat 2 tablespoons of olive oil in a large skillet. Add onions and sauté for 1 minute.

Now, add in ground beef and sauté for an additional minutes, stirring constantly. Stir in mushrooms stems, tomatoes, bell pepper, salt, and black pepper, and continue to sauté for a further 3 minutes.

Arrange mushroom caps on a clean work surface and drizzle with the remaining oil. Scoop the beef mixture into each cap and place in a large vacuum-sealable bag in a single layer. Release air by the water displacement method, seal and submerge the bag in the water bath. Set the timer for 50 minutes.

Once the timer has stopped, remove the mushrooms from the bag. Transfer to a serving dish. Pour over any of the mushroom juices that are left in bag. Serve with salad.

Classic Beef Stew

Prep + Cook Time: 3 hours 15 minutes | Servings: 4

Ingredients:

1 pound beef neck, chopped into bite-sized pieces

½ large eggplant, sliced

1 cup fire-roasted tomatoes

1 cup beef broth

½ cup burgundy

¼ cup vegetable oil

5 peppercorns, whole

2 tbsp butter, unsalted

1 bay leaf, whole

1 tbsp tomato paste

½ tbsp cayenne pepper

¼ tsp chili pepper (optional)

1 tsp salt

Fresh parsley to garnish

Directions:

Prepare a water bath and place the Sous Vide in it. Set to 135 F. Rinse the meat under cold running water. Pat dry with a kitchen paper and place on a clean working surface. Using a sharp knife, cut into bite-sized pieces.

In a large bowl, combine burgundy with oil, peppercorns, bay leaf, cayenne pepper, chili pepper, and salt. Dip meat in this mixture and refrigerate for 2 hours. Remove the meat from the marinade and pat dry with a kitchen paper. Reserve the liquid. Place in a large vacuum-sealable bag. Seal the bag.

Submerge the sealed bag in the water bath and cook for 1 hour. Remove from the water bath, discard the bay leaf, and transfer to a deep, heavy-bottomed pot. Add butter and gently melt over medium heat. Put in eggplants, tomatoes, and ¼ cup of the marinade. Cook for a further 5 minutes, stirring constantly. Taste, adjust the seasonings and serve garnished with chopped fresh parsley.

Garlic Burgers

Prep + Cook Time: 70 minutes | Servings: 4

Ingredients:

1 pound lean ground beef

3 garlic cloves, crushed

2 tbsp breadcrumbs

3 eggs, beaten

4 burger buns

4 crisphead lettuce leaves

4 tomato slices

¼ cup lentils, soaked

¼ cup oil, divided in half

1 tbsp cilantro, finely chopped

Salt and black pepper to taste

Directions:

Prepare a water bath, place Sous Vide in it, and set to 139 F.

Meanwhile, in a bowl, combine lentils with beef, garlic, cilantro, breadcrumbs, eggs, and three tablespoons of oil. Season with salt and black pepper. Using your hands, shape burgers and lay on a lightly floured working surface. Gently place each burger in a vacuum-sealable bag and seal. Submerge in the water bath and cook for 1 hour.

Once the timer has stopped, carefully remove the burgers from the bag and pat them dry with paper towel. Set aside. Heat up the remaining oil in a large skillet. Brown burgers for 2-3 minutes on each side for extra crispiness. Drizzle burgers with your favorite sauce and transfer to buns. Garnish as with lettuce and tomato and serve immediately.

Ground Beef Stew

Prep + Cook Time: 60 minutes | Servings: 3

Ingredients:

4 medium-sized eggplants, halved

½ cup lean ground beef

2 medium-size tomatoes, chopped

¼ cup extra virgin olive oil

2 tbsp toasted almonds, finely chopped

1 tbsp fresh celery leaves, finely chopped

Salt and black pepper to taste

1 tsp thyme

Directions:

Prepare a water bath and place the Sous Vide in it. Set to 180 F. Slice eggplants in half, lengthwise. Scoop the flesh and transfer to a bowl. Generously sprinkle with salt and let sit for ten minutes.

Heat up 3 tablespoons of oil over medium heat. Briefly fry the eggplants, for 3 minutes on each side and remove from the frying pan. Use some kitchen paper to soak up the excess oil. Set aside.

Put in ground beef to the same frying pan. Stir-fry for 5 minutes, stir in tomatoes and simmer until the tomatoes have softened. Add in eggplants, almonds and celery leaves and cook for 5 minutes. Turn off heat and stir in thyme.

Transfer everything to a large vacuum-sealable bag. Release air by the water displacement method, seal and submerge the bag in the water bath. Set the timer for 40 minutes.

Once the timer has stopped, remove the bag and pour the contents over a large bowl. Taste and adjust the seasonings. Serve garnished with parsley, if desired.

Beef Sirloin in Tomato Sauce

Prep + Cook Time: 2 hours 5 minutes | Servings: 3

Ingredients:

1 pound beef sirloin medallions

1 cup fire-roasted tomatoes

1 tsp hot pepper sauce

3 garlic cloves, crushed

2 tsp chili pepper

2 tsp garlic powder

2 tsp fresh lime juice

1 bay leaf

2 tsp vegetable oil

Salt and black pepper to taste

Directions:

Prepare a water bath, place Sous Vide in it, and set to 129 F. Season beef with salt and black pepper.

In a bowl, combine the fire roasted tomatoes with hot pepper sauce, crushed garlic, chili pepper, garlic powder, and lime juice. Add the sirloin to the mixture and toss to coat. Place in the vacuum-sealable bag in a single layer and seal it. Submerge in the water bath and cook for 2 hours.

Once the timer has stopped, remove the medallions and pat them dry. Discard the bay leaf. Reserve cooking juices. Sear in a high hot skillet about 1 minute. Serve with the sauce and mashed potatoes.

Beef with Onions

Prep + Cook Time: 1 hour 15 minutes | Servings: 3

Ingredients:

¾ cup lean beef, s chopped into bite-sized pieces

2 large onions, peeled and finely chopped

¼ cup water

3 tbsp mustard

1 tsp soy sauce

1 tsp dried thyme

2 tbsp vegetable oil

2 tbsp sesame oil

Directions:

Prepare a water bath and place the Sous Vide in it. Set to 136 F. Rinse the meat and pat dry with a kitchen paper. Using a kitchen brush, spread the mustard over meat and sprinkle with dried thyme.

Place in a vacuum-sealable bag along with soy sauce, chopped onions, and sesame oil. Seal the bag. and submerge in the bath and cook for 1 hour. Remove from the water bath. Pat the meat dry with a paper towel and set aside.

Heat the vegetable oil in a large skillet, over medium heat. Add beef chops and stir-fry for 5 minutes, stirring constantly. Remove from the heat and serve.

Garlicky Prime Ribs

Prep + Cook Time: 10 hours 15 minutes | Servings: 8

Ingredients:

3 pounds prime rib, trimmed

1 rosemary sprig

1 thyme sprig

Salt and black pepper to taste

6 garlic cloves

1 tbsp olive oil

Directions:

Prepare a water bath and place the Sous Vide in it. Set to 140 F. Season the rib with salt and pepper and place it in a vacuum-sealable bag with thyme and rosemary. Release air by the water displacement method, seal and submerge the bag in water bath. Set the timer for 10 hours.

Once the timer has stopped, remove the bag. Crush the garlic cloves into a paste, spread the paste over the meat. Heat the olive oil in a pan and sear the meat on all sides, for a few minutes.

Beef Fillet with Baby Carrots

Prep + Cook Time: 2 hours 15 minutes | Servings: 5

Ingredients:

2 pounds beef fillet

7 baby carrots, sliced

1 onion, chopped

1 cup tomato paste

2 tbsp vegetable oil

2 tbsp fresh parsley, finely chopped

Salt and black pepper to taste

Directions:

Prepare a water bath and place the Sous Vide in it. Set to 133 F. Wash and pat dry the meat with a kitchen paper. Using a sharp knife, cut into bite-sized pieces and season with salt and pepper.

In a skillet, brown beef in oil over medium heat, turning to brown equally for 5 minutes.

Now, add sliced carrots and onion to the skillet, cooking until softened, about 2 minutes. Stir in tomato paste, salt, and pepper. Pour in ½ cup of water.

Remove from the heat and transfer to a large vacuum-sealable bag in a single layer. Release air by the water displacement method, seal and submerge the bag in the water bath. Set the timer for 2 hours. Remove the bag from the bath and transfer contents to serving plate. Serve garnished with fresh parsley.

Red Wine Beef Ribs

Prep + Cook Time: 6 hours 15 minutes | Servings: 3

Ingredients:

1 pound beef short ribs

¼ cup red wine

1 tsp honey

½ cup tomato paste

2 tbsp olive oil

½ cup beef stock

¼ cup apple cider vinegar

1 garlic clove, minced

1 tsp Paprika

Salt and black pepper to taste

Directions:

Prepare a water bath and place the Sous Vide in it. Set to 140 F. Rinse and drain the ribs. Season with salt, pepper, and paprika. Place in a vacuum-sealable bag in a single layer along with wine, tomato paste, beef broth, honey, and apple cider. Release air by the water displacement method, seal and submerge the bag in the water bath. Set the timer for 6 hours. Pat the ribs dry. Discard cooking liquids.

In a large skillet, heat up the olive oil over medium heat. Add garlic and stir-fry until translucent. Put in ribs and brown for 5 minutes per side.

Beef Pepper Meat

Prep + Cook Time: 6 hours 10 minutes | Servings: 2

Ingredients:

1 pound beef tenderloin, cut into bite-sized pieces

1 large onion finely chopped

1 tbsp butter, melted

1 tbsp fresh parsley, finely chopped

1 tsp dried thyme, ground

1 tbsp lemon juice, freshly squeezed

1 tbsp tomato paste

Salt and black pepper to taste

Directions:

Prepare a water bath and place the Sous Vide in it. Set to 158 F. Thoroughly combine all the ingredients, except for the parsley, in a large vacuum-sealable bag. Release air by the water displacement method, seal and submerge the bag in the water bath. Set the timer for 6 hours.

Once the timer has stopped, remove from the water bath and open the bag. Serve immediately garnished with chopped fresh parsley.

Beef Stroganoff

Prep + Cook Time: 24 hours 15 minutes | Servings: 4

Ingredients:

1 pound chuck roast, cut into chunks

½ onion, chopped

1 pound mushrooms, sliced

1 garlic cloves, minced

¼ cup white wine

4 tbsp Greek yogurt

½ cup beef stock

1 tbsp butter

1 sprig of fresh flat-leaf parsley

Salt and black pepper to taste

Directions:

Prepare a water bath and place the Sous Vide in it. Set to 140 F. Season the beef with salt and pepper. Place in a vacuum-sealable bag and seal. Immerse in the preheated water and cook for 24 hours.

The next day, melt the butter in a pan over medium heat. Put in onions and garlic and sauté until softened, about 3 minutes. Add in mushrooms and cook for an additional 5 minutes. Pour in wine and stock and cook until the mixture is reduced by half.

Stir in the beef and cook for another minute. Taste and adjust the seasonings. Serve warm with minced fresh parsley.

Beef Bites with Teriyaki Sauce & Seeds

Prep + Cook Time: 70 minutes | Servings: 2

I ngredients

2 beef steaks

½ cup teriyaki sauce

2 tbsp soy sauce

2 tsp fresh chilis, chopped

1½ tbsp sesame seeds, toasted

2 tbsp poppy seeds, toasted

8 oz rice noodles

2 tbsp sesame oil

1 tbsp scallion, finely chopped

Di rections

Prepare a water bath and place the Sous Vide in it. Set to 134 F. Chop the beef in cubes and place in a vacuum-sealable bag. Add 1/2 cup of teriyaki sauce. Release air by the water displacement method, seal and submerge the bag in the water bath. Cook for 60 minutes.

In a bowl, mix the soy sauce and chilis. In another bowl, put the poppy seeds. After 50 minutes, start cooking the noodles. Drain them and transfer to a bowl. Once the timer has stopped, remove the beef and discard cooking juices. Heat the sesame oil in a skillet over high heat and add in beef with 6 tbsp of teriyaki sauce. Cook for 5 seconds. Serve in a bowl and garnish with toasted seeds.

Lemony & Peppery Flank Steak

Prep + Cook Time: 2 hours 15 minutes | Servings: 4

Ingredients:

2 pounds flank steak

1 tbsp lime zest

1 lemon, sliced

½ tsp cayenne pepper

1 tsp garlic powder

Salt and black pepper to taste

¼ cup maple syrup

½ cup chicken stock

Directions:

Prepare a water bath and place the Sous Vide in it. Set to 148 F. Combine the spices and zest and rub over the steak. Let sit for about 5 minutes.

Whisk the stock and maple syrup. Place the steak in a vacuum-sealable bag and add the lemon slices. Release air by the water displacement method, seal and submerge the bag in water bath. Set timer for 2 hours. Once done, remove and transfer to a grill and cook for 30 seconds each side. Serve immediately.

Beef & Veggie Stew

Prep + Cook Time: 4 hours 25 minutes | Servings: 12

Ingredients:

16 ounces beef fillet, cubed

4 potatoes, chopped

3 carrots, sliced

5 ounces shallot, sliced

1 onion, chopped

2 garlic cloves, minced

¼ cup red wine

¼ cup heavy cream

2 tbsp butter

1 tsp paprika

½ cup chicken stock

½ tsp turmeric

Salt and black pepper to taste

1 tsp lemon juice

Directions:

Prepare a water bath and place the Sous Vide in it. Set to 155 F. Place the beef along with salt, pepper, turmeric, paprika, and red wine in a vacuum-sealable bag. Massage to coat well. Release air by the water displacement method, seal and submerge the bag in water bath. Set the timer for 4 hours.

Meanwhile, combine the remaining ingredients in another vacuum-sealable bag. Seal and immerse it in the same bath 3 hours before the end of the cooking time of the meat. Once done, remove everything and place in a pot over medium heat and cook for 15 minutes.

Honey-Dijon Brisket

Prep + Cook Time: 48 hours 20 minutes | Servings: 12

Ingredients

6 pounds beef brisket

2 tbsp olive oil

4 large shallots, sliced

4 garlic cloves, peeled and smashed

¼ cup apple cider vinegar

½ cup tomato paste

½ cup honey

¼ cup Dijon mustard

2 cups water

1 tbsp whole black peppercorns

2 dried allspice berries

Salt to taste

Directions

Prepare a water bath and place the Sous Vide in it. Set to 155 F.

Heat the olive oil in a skillet over high heat and sear the brisket until golden brown both sides. Set aside. In the same skillet on medium heat sauté shallots and garlic for 10 minutes.

Combine vinegar, honey, tomato paste, mustard, peppercorn, water, allspice, and cloves. Add in the shallot mixture. Mix well. Place the brisket and the mixture in a vacuum-sealable bag. Release air by the water displacement method, seal and submerge the bag in the water bath. Cook for 48 hours.

Once the timer has stopped, remove the bag and pat the meat dry. Pour the cooking juices in a saucepan over high heat and cook until the sauce has reduced by half, 10 minutes. Serve with the brisket.

Rosemary Ribeye Stew

Prep + Cook Time: 6 hours 35 minutes | Servings: 12

Ingredients

3 pounds bone-in beef ribeye roast

Salt and black pepper to taste

1 tbsp green pepper

1 tbsp dried celery seeds

2 tbsp garlic powder

4 sprigs rosemary

1 tbsp cumin

1 cup beef stock

2 egg whites

Directions

Marinate the beef with salt. Allow chilling for 12 hours. Prepare a water bath and place the Sous Vide in it. Set to 132 F. Place the beef in a vacuum-sealable bag. Release air by the water displacement method, seal and submerge the bag in the water bath. Cook for 6 hours.

Preheat the oven to 425 F. Once the timer has stopped, remove the beef and pat dry. Combine peppers, celery seeds, garlic powder, cumin, and rosemary. Drizzle the roasted beef with a white egg, celery mixture and salt. Place the roast in a baking tray and bake for 10 minutes. Allow cooling for 10 minutes and slice. Plate the beef and top with the sauce.

Divine Sirloin with Sweet Potato Purée

Prep + Cook Time: 1 hour 20 minutes | Servings: 4

Ingredients

4 sirloin steaks

2 pounds sweet potatoes, cubed

¼ cup steak seasoning

Salt and black pepper to taste

4 tbsp butter

Canola oil for searing

Directions

Prepare a water bath and place the Sous Vide in it. Set to 129 F. Place the seasoned steaks in a vacuum-sealable bag. Release air by the water displacement method, seal and submerge the bag in the water bath. Cook for 1 hour.

Boil the potatoes for 15 minutes. Drain it and transfer to a bowl with butter. Mash and season with salt and pepper. Once the timer has stopped, remove the steaks and pat dry. Heat the oil in a pot over medium heat. Sear for 1 minute. Serve with the potato puree.

Beef Pie with Mushrooms

Prep + Cook Time: 2 hours 40 minutes | Servings: 4

Ingredients

1 pound beef tenderloin fillet

Salt and black pepper to taste

2 tbsp Dijon mustard

1 sheet puff pastry, thawed

8 oz cremini mushrooms

8 oz shiitake mushrooms

1 shallot, diced

3 cloves garlic, chopped

1 tbsp butter

6 slices bacon

Directions

Prepare a water bath and place the Sous Vide in it. Set to 124 F. Season the beef with salt and pepper and place in a vacuum-sealable bag. Release air by the water displacement method, seal and submerge the bag in the water bath. Cook for 2 hours. Put the mushrooms in a food processor and pulse.

In a hot skillet cook shallots and garlic, when tender add in mushrooms and cook until the water has evaporated. Add 1 tbsp of butter and cook. Once the timer has stopped, remove the beef and pat dry.

Heat oil in a skillet over medium heat and sear the beef for 30 seconds each side. Brush the beef with Dijon mustard. In a plastic foil, arrange prosciutto slices and bacon. Place beef on top. Roll them and allow chilling for 20 minutes. Roll out the puff pastry and brush with egg. Put beef inside. Heat the oven to 475 F and bake for 10 minutes. Slice and serve.

CPSIA information can be obtained
at www.ICGtesting.com
Printed in the USA
LVHW080701030521
686315LV00009B/177